STRESS, BURNOUT, AND ADDICTION IN THE NURSING PROFESSION

STRESS, BURNOUT, AND ADDICTION IN THE NURSING PROFESSION

HERBERT R. WARNER PH.D

To order additional copies of this book, contact:
Xlibris LLC
1-888-795-4274
www.Xlibris.com
Orders@Xlibris.com
552201

CONTENTS

PART THREE
Addiction Section

Acknowledgments

FIRST AND FOREMOST, I want to thank the universal God for giving me the wisdom and the energy to complete this book. I also would like to acknowledge him for giving me the desire to help people while on this life journey. I want to thank my lovely wife, Hortencia (*mi corazon*), for her support during late nights of writing. I would like to thank all the people who have encouraged me to finish this project. I would like to acknowledge all the nurses I interviewed about their experiences as a nurse and all the RNs who made a contribution with their input and opinions. I would like to thank all the people at Xlibris who helped me with this book project. I am grateful to them for their guidance and advice.

Stress, Burnout, and Addiction in the Nursing Profession

There are some jobs in which it is impossible for a man [or woman] to be virtuous.

—Aristotle (384-322 BC)

INTRODUCTION

BENEATH THE BEAUTIFUL decorated scrubs, jackets, shirts, caps, and colorful nursing uniforms are people who are tired, worn out, stressed, and burned out. They are mothers, fathers, girlfriends, boyfriends, and students who are gainfully employed and working to provide for their families and to further their education and career growth. When you think about a nurse, you picture a beautiful person, caring, compassionate, sometimes sexy, but that is not always the case. Some wear a mask to cover or hide the results from stress, burnout, and addictions that they have encountered during their journey in the health-care arena. Health-care reform was one of the themes of the Obama administration, with its billions of dollars' cost, which still has not been fully implemented; they failed to address the cost of fallout from overworked, stressed-out, and addicted RNs in the health-care field.

Nurses regularly hear the phrases, "You are a great nurse," "Hang in there," "Good job," "Nice call," and you keep telling yourself, "I am OK. I love my job," and crying most of the time, knowing very well that things are not going to change but will stay the same. Such praise can actually contribute to burnout. "If someone says you are doing great, then you feel like you must keep going, and the real deal is, you don't have to. When are the powers to be going to triage this "bloody mess" of stress, burnout, and addiction with our frontline emergency medical staff? Where are our top medical and mental-health managers and administrators of hospitals? What are they doing? You answer the question. We spend billions of dollars on our nation's defense by purchasing weapons of mass destruction to fight a proposed war on terror. However, we cannot give a small fraction of percent to help fund our mental-health programs. Finally, the government is talking about making mental-health practitioners a part of a larger network of insurance providers that get reimbursed for their services. They now realize that mental-health issues are a disease that must be treated like any other medical problems. But we had to wait to have a tragedy like Sandy Hook Elementary, where twenty innocent children and six adults lost lives. President Obama believes it is a gun-control problem, and I agree to some extent, but I would add also that it is a mental-health control problem. We as a nation have not given proper attention and funding to our mental-health population. People who have mentally diagnosed diseases are being released from institutions on conditional releases and restricted releases. This is not the solution to the mental-health problems or a solution to the person who is being treated for a mental diagnosis. Our state mental-health hospitals and local behavioral-health providers are not well managed or operated properly; money is thrown at these institutions, and they are left to manage themselves with little oversight. Government needs to pay attention to this issue and act responsible and fund these areas. Obama administration suggests allocating $10 million for research on the causes of gun violence; we need more research in the causes of violence offenders who have some sort of mental disorder. RNs are on the front line, along with counselors, who see and administer care and administer drug treatment; it is the RN who must be attentive and vigilant to properly care for this population. They are the ones who must treat these psychotic, delusional, and depressed people. Therefore, our medical staff that serves you and me and the general public must also serve the mentally ill population; so in the following chapters, we will talk about and discuss stress, burnout, and addiction as it pertains to RNs working in the health-care industry. It is a problem in our cities, state, and country that no one has properly addressed this issue, at least not for any extended period of time. There has not been any funding in the way of education, seminars, treatment, and retraining given to our RN and to schools and universities that train our nurses. It is about time someone draws attention to this vital important issue in our country. When there is an emergency with our family, child, partner, friend, or loved one, we go to the nearest emergency department, clinic, or hospital to seek help. We expect that the person or persons caring for our loved one are competent, alert, attentive, and ready to perform the duties that they were trained for; but if the RN and staff are burned out, stressed, and have some type of addiction, it is very unlikely you or your loved one will get the attention and treatment they deserve and need. This is an emergency. Someone needs to call 911 for our health-care industry. In the following chapters, I will discuss the cause and effect of stress, burnout, and addiction as it relates to our RNs that work in our hospitals, emergency rooms, and clinics. My hope is that this book will shed some light on an industry that is in need of an overhaul to its methods of operations and its administrators. It is my desire that each person who works as a nurse will consider what this book has to say about stress, burnout, and addiction. It is also my desire that each person who comes to a clinic, hospital, or an emergency room would have the care they deserve and need during a time of crisis. We need to take a serious look at our frontline medical personnel. Also, let me say that I know there are great, smart, caring, and wonderful RNs who are not addicted or burned out and do a great job of taking care of people who are injured and sick, and need their services at the emergency room or hospitals. The truth is no matter how great you are, no matter how well you function, there is stress in all of our lives, and sometimes it gets the best of us. I want everyone to give credit to where credit is due—to all the RNs who do an amazing job; but also please get help for the RNs who need it and help to the one who is hiding it, denying it, and who don't know how to ask for it.

PART ONE

STRESS

CHAPTER ONE

Viral—It's In the Air

Stress is when you wake up screaming and
realize you haven't fallen asleep yet.

—Unknown

NO ONE IS immune from stress; it affects the executive, and it affects the homeless person, the poor and the rich, and the good and the bad. You see, stress has no respect for person. You can be walking in the supermarket and cannot decide on which soup to buy because there are so many, and stress will attack your mind. There is nothing to fight; it is not something physical but a state of mind. It is like there is something in the air; it is changing our world in which we live, and it is changing the workplace. You ever wonder why the workplace is becoming so violent? Well, people are stressed, have no patience, are on edge, or are angry at something, and the end result is they become violent. The nature of work is changing at a whirlwind speed. Perhaps now more than ever before, job stress poses a threat to the health of workers and, in turn, to the health organizations. Job requirements are very demanding; there are more duties and details than ever before. On the job, stress is increasing. Job stress is the harmful physical and emotional responses that occur when one's body and mind cannot match the capabilities, resources, or needs of the job. Job stress can lead to poor health and even injury. Many people visit emergency rooms each day for stress—and work-related symptoms. The symptoms can be as small as not having the ability to think properly to a sudden loss of memory and to the classic panic attacks, which are caused by, in most cases, increased stressors. Peoples are being treated at an alarming rate each day in our emergency rooms for one or more of these types of stressors.

Every year, there are thousands of people who work themselves to death. People are working long hours without taking a break; they are missing lunch breaks or will just not eat lunch—all because of the demands of the job and sometimes just to please a boss or supervisor who do not care too much about you other than making sure you do a good job. The trend today is to hire fewer than adequate staff and work them to the maximum limits. And the results and the stress aren't limited to any one level of employee. It affects upper management, staff on frontlines, and nursing assistance. It affects across the board even down to the janitor. Now managers have more responsibilities and must produce more. Nurse managers, who usually supervise only eight or nine nurses, are now managing three to four times that many; and at some hospitals, six to eight times as many. The increased duties are causing stress and burnout. Unfortunately, there's very little organizations can do about the global and economic conditions requiring leaner staffs, but there are many actions that can lessen the impact of stress and burnout. We will explore those actions later in the preceding chapters on how to manage stress and burnout.

You must remember, nurses are special people and have needs just like everyone else; it is no less difficult being a nurse as it is becoming a nurse. Nursing school is challenging, and the vicissitudes of the job experience can be emotionally draining. Most students do not expect much stress in nursing; they think it is all about taking care of people's needs and giving them medicine and everyone is OK. Well, everyone is not OK; in fact, RNs have more challenges today than ever before: high-tech computer charting, leaner staff, micromanagers, issues with management, and hostile patients. And the list goes on and on, until you find a nurse in trouble with addiction, stress, or burnout. You see, most people are too preoccupied with their sickness and their own well-being around nurses to think about how the nurse feels.

It is not uncommon for nurses to experience "stress and burnout." They spend a short time with many patients, and the patients are always in a state of crisis or just not being well. It becomes difficult to experience or form relationships with people in these conditions. Another reason is time spent with them; you are constantly being rushed and told by your charge nurse, "Get them out as soon as possible," because they need that bed and people are lining up in the waiting room. The RN has this constant pressure to perform their jobs quickly. Some people do not operate very well under pressure, but a nurse must learn to do exactly that—perform under pressure. The good news is that nursing is a very rewarding and noble career. Nurses must keep in mind that people are mainly concerned for their own welfare when they come to an ER during these situations, and they are heavily dependent on nurses taking care of them and providing them with reassurance and telling them that they will be all right.

Nursing the Nurse

When you live next to the cemetery,
you can't cry for everyone who dies.
> —Russian Proverb

MOST OF US, whether we are professional helpers or not, tend to personalize too much. We absorb the sadness, anxiety, and negativity of those around us. Sometimes we even feel this is expected of us . . . As we listen to stories of terrible things that happen (or observe them), we catch some of their futility, fear, vulnerability, and hopelessness rather than experiencing mere frustration or concern. We learn that no matter how professionally prepared we are, we are not immune to the psychological and spiritual dangers that arise in living a full life of involvement with others. RNs have extended family assigned to them each day and don't even realize it. They care for them, listen to stories, absorb anxiety, and try to make people's situation better, even though they barely know them.

RNs who have worked in the field for years typically tell the same stories of issues in their own lives that describe a relationship or marriage gone wrong or destroyed from lack of time put into the marriage, or affairs that happen on the job, or about many types of addictions, betrayal, no support from management, and the list goes on. So what do you do when you have done all you can and that's still not enough? That is the sentiment of many health-care workers, especially RNs all around the world; it is not just limited to your little city. Now let's us look more into stress in the next chapter and see how it affects your job, marriage, children, extended family, and actually your whole entire being.

Chapter Two

Feeling Stress-say

Any idiot can face a crisis—it's this day-to-day living that wears you out.

—Anton Chekhov

STRESS IS A fact of life—for mostly every human on this planet—a harsh reality that must be dealt with. Stress is so popular that other people are offended if we don't appear to be under stress ourselves. They will say to you, "What is the matter with you?" They want you to worry about something, and if you are not worrying or stressing, they want to know what your problem is. Stress is a constant, ever-going, and ever-pressing stimulus that ponders your mind with what-ifs, why not, what happened, how can I? Stress is seen as a necessary part of achievement, relationships, careers, and life. The word has become a universal catchall to describe, validate, and explain everything that is wrong in our lives. "I am just feeling a little stressed"; it is what we hear all the time from our friends, loved ones, and coworkers. We live in a world of smartphones, laptops, Twitter, and Facebook. We have connections to anything or anyone in a matter of seconds, and yet we are stressed, constantly watching our phones and sending text messages. We play our little games on the

phone, yet we are stressed beyond belief. It's not like we don't know where the other person is or what he or she is doing; we know every minute! You will get an alert or posting on your Facebook page!

"I'm stressed out." What does that really mean? "I am feeling stressed." So what is the definition of stress? In my opinion, stress is the pressures we feel from life, how we perceive it, how we believe what we feel, how we react to it, and how we cope with these tensions and pressures of life.

People often make this quote: "If I weren't under so much stress, my life would be better"; I would feel much better is a very common belief indeed. It is how we define our lives now on how we feel.

Stress is a major cause of unrest in our lives; by that, I mean we as a society do not get enough rest or sleep. I believe sleep deprivation is a major cause of stress; when we don't get enough sleep, our bodies do not react properly. There are more mistakes with medications; if you work as an RN and don't get enough sleep, you forget to do a report or give the wrong lab value to the doctor, but we don't have to surrender our lives to being overworked. There comes a stopping point in one's life where we say enough is enough—"I am going to take care of myself."

Accidents happen; suddenly, unexplained, unexpected events happen in our lives, and pow! We are instantly stressed out! You often hear people say, "Don't talk to me, I have an emergency" or "I have to go, bye." Author Dr. Richard Carlson said, "Stress is nothing more than a socially acceptable form of mental illness." I would not go as far as to put that label on stress, but I would say it is close to describing the craziest that stress can cause in one's life. People make the wrong decision when under stress; some people refuse to make decisions or choices while under stress, whereas some people hurt themselves while under stress. Some people do really dumb things while "stressed out." So where do we put it? Define it?

The moment we define stress as coming from anywhere other than from within ourselves, we are in denial.

We know that depression, stress, and addiction can affect anyone at any time. It is the everyday stuff that happens to us that is the bottom line. But as health professionals, we are often very busy caring for our patients, and we don't take time to care for ourselves or realize colleagues maybe in need of care themselves. High levels of stress, burnout, and addiction often strike nurses and anyone in the nursing profession. It is well recognized that many nurses and nursing assistants experience fatigue, which affects their health and safety.

Often people won't talk about how they are feeling or acknowledge they may be feeling unwell. For nurses and nursing assistants, it is particularly difficult for some to go from being the one who cares for people to being the one cared for, and this can prevent them from seeking assistance. It is the very nature of the way the nursing profession works that can eventually catch up with them. Several systems of rotating shifts from days to nights, heavy workloads, and difficulties with sleep patterns; family-life commitments and more work responsibilities and less time to carry out these duties take their toll. Anecdotally, we know nurses take less care of themselves—for example, not taking lunch breaks when it is busy, writing patients' clinical notes long after the shift has finished. This can sometimes create a very unhealthy habit that results in anxiety, stress, burnout, and addiction.

CHAPTER THREE

Workplace Stress

The best index to a person's character is how he or she treats people who can't fight back.
—Abigail Van Buren

IT IS THE responsibility of all nurses (RN) to look out for each other, and if we recognize the symptoms of stress, depression, burnout, and addiction in a colleague, we must try and help them seek assistance. It is important for all of us to involve ourselves in good support systems, whether that support is at work, home, or within a family member. It is also vital to have activities that you really enjoy undertaking outside of working hours. This helps to take your mind away from work and the pressures you may feel at work. If you think you are becoming so bogged down by work pressures, do yourself a favor and speak to someone about it. Think about your health physically, emotionally, and spiritually, and make choices about how you are going to look after yourself.

The average nurse is experiencing so much workplace stress that they are having mental breakdowns and requiring interventions at a higher rate than seen in years. When I worked in the ER, it was the social worker's duties and responsibility to counsel and give support to the RN in their time of personal crisis. I can safety estimate that I only talked to about three or four nurses during an entire year. Now, that was seven or eight years ago. Now it is reported that nurses have increased their visits to counselors and management requesting time off for personal crisis. The health-care industry and hospital staff stress have changed in severity and causes; one is because of the economic downturn, and nurses are scared of losing their jobs. Nurses have a small margin for mistakes; the fear of write-ups, warning, license being suspended, and dismissal is always present. When nurses have to deal with management is one thing, but dealing with these nursing boards because of an incident or someone accused you falsely is a totally different animal. This is one thing that pushes an RN stress to a different level. Another thing that increases workplace stress is that nurses are not taking vacations, they are not taking lunches, they are not taking breaks, plus they are working a lot of overtime and double shifts. Sound familiar? "Can you stay an extra three hours or just cover the shift?" One stressor too many happens, and it's the straw that breaks the camel's back.

Well, one may ask what behaviors are reported more than others. There are three types of behaviors reported more than others; you may be surprised to hear them. After talking with several different nurses, they reported violence, hallucinations, and suicidal comments. Yes, in the workplace, you have these types of behaviors; problem is that they are not reported! These types of behavior can immediately get you fired, suspended, or referred to HR. Most nurses do not use their EAP (Employee Assistance Program); remember, employees' health and well-being are the newest buzzwords in corporate America, with most companies working feverishly to integrate wellness programs in their work cultures. It is clear to all that workplace stress, apart from employee health habits—or a lack of them—is a significant reason for the growing prevalence of lifestyle diseases such as diabetes, heart disease, obesity, and hypertension. RNs are familiar with signing bonuses; nothing motivates like money does, and so health-care companies have started realizing that the easiest way to entice staff into wellness program is to use money as an incentive. This is a proactive approach because wellness initiative often generates great interest, provided the themes are tweaked in keeping with the corporate values and specific needs so they will not be seen in any negative way. Everyone realizes that there is a correlation between cardiovascular disease, depression, burnout, and stress. Chronic job stress is strongly associated with violent, being overweight, or obese. These are employees like executives, police officers, and RN, for example, that work long hours, do not eat well, or do not exercise. In especially stressful times, they resort to chocolate, junk food, coffees, and energy drinks— OMG! Even the kids are drinking an energy drink, go figure! Kids mimic their parents. They watch you and notice how you handle crisis and how you deal with situations. And of course, some resort to using drugs.

WORK HARD—PLAY HARD

I have heard more nurses use this quote than any other: "Work hard— play hard." Well, let me ask the question, "How has that worked out for you?" I can honestly say from talking and interviewing several nurses, it has not worked out very well; they have reported divorces, family dysfunction, spousal abuse, problems with their children, alcohol addictions, drug addiction, and the list goes on. Remember what I said about sleep deprivation in the previous chapter? When the body does not get the proper rest and sleep it needs, it leads to stress, and stress leads to arguments, violent, divorce, and addictions. When you work hard and play hard, you have no time for sleep.

We have a stress epidemic in our nation. The majority of Americans very likely have excessive stress in their lives, and constant reports of stress seem to indicate that the percentage of Americans each year who feel under "a great deal of stress" is rising.

According to Don Colbert, MD, "90 percent of all visits to your PCP (primary care physician) office are stress disorders and that Americans are consuming five billion tranquilizers, five billion barbiturates, and sixteen tons of aspirin." Wow! So why are people still depressed and stressed out? Because doctors and nurses are treating the symptoms, not the disease! Whenever you feel bad or down, take a pill, and it all will go away— wrong! Several housewives became addicted to prescription pills by taking that advice. How many of the housewives were nurses? These drugs do not prevent stress. There are serious doubts about medication's ability to treat stress in the first place. It is sad to say, but nurses are very moody. And at times, a nurse can very easily masquerade a mood disorder with a physical problem or sleep deprivation. I would say about one in five working aged Americans, including RNs, experience symptoms of a mental-health disorder in any given month, be it depression, anxiety, or addiction-type problems, which are among the most common.

Because of the stigma associated with psychiatric disorders, RNs may be reluctant to seek treatment, especially in the current economic climate, when they are concerned about losing their jobs. At the same time, nurse managers may want to help but might not know where to start. As a result, mental-health problems in our medical world often go undetected and untreated for years. Or until we hear of a tragedy where a health-care worker kills several people or commits suicide. Then you will hear the question, what are we doing to help our nurses? I believe it is better to be proactive now and not have regrets later. Our frontline medical nursing staff needs help and, in most cases, treatment and rehab. However, it is not a quick fix, but definitely beneficial in the long term of a company and its employee.

Let's look into what would cause stress in our RN or medical staff.

THESE ARE THE MAJOR CATEGORIES THAT PRODUCE STRESS:

TABLE 1

Major life stressors:
1   Divorce or separation
2   Death in the family
3   Serious illness you have or a loved one has
4   Not having enough money
5   You are not happy in your job or workplace.
6   Relationship issues with your partner
7   Marriage problems
8   Addiction issues

Less major (everyday stuff)
1   Stuck in traffic
2   Paying bills on time
3   Problems with your children

4   Cell phone broke
5   Sexuality
6   Sleep deprivation
7   Phobias
7   Holiday shopping

Let's look into a little more detail.

COMMON STRESSORS:

TABLE 2

1   **Physical stress:** Sleep deprivation often arises from lack of sleep, overworking, working extra shifts and days, excessive exercise, trying to get that perfect figure, physical injury or trauma, or broken arm or leg, which makes everyday routine difficult.
2   **Emotional and mental stress:** (a) Various emotions such as anger, especially at your boss for his or her decision; (b) hostility in the workplace, having bullies yelling at you; and (c) depression, anxiety, and fear, not knowing the outcome of a situation (test or exam), can cause chronic emotional stress. The same for mental stress: the worries and general anxiety that often arise from too much and too little play, too much debt, marital difficulties, children using drugs or alcohol, failing in school, and, of course, other mental stresses.
2   **Chemical stress:** Comes from excessive use of various substances such as energy drinks with excessive sugar, your favorite coffee shops with lattes, double shots of caffeine, stimulants, alcohol, nicotine—smoking your favorite cigarette—and all of the many food additives.

CHAPTER FOUR

Can Your Words Cause Stress?

*Words are like delicate feathers . . . Once you release them in the
wind, you cannot retrieve them.*

—Wise Priest

WE HAVE HEARD it said to us: "Sticks and stone may break my bones, but words will never hurt me." Wrong! The impact of your words—yes, words—can hurt! It can come from your supervisor or your coworker; something as simple as words can have a traumatic impact on us and induce stress in our lives. Think back to a time when someone said some harsh words to you. Whether they were true or not, they had an effect on you. Words can build you up, and words can tear you down. When we let things people say to us affect us, we are setting ourselves up for stress. When we continue to play these words over in our heads, and then rewind them again and again, we create stress within our minds and start a cycle of helplessness. Remember, you are not what someone says about you. In the medical field, and especially nursing, you hear a lot of negative, condescending, vulgar words, and sometimes they are directly toward you. And it is how you react to these words that determine the emotional effect it will have on you.

Some of us are terribly affected when our supervisors say something negative or just say something vague; we worry and stress out because we are concerned that we did something wrong and our boss is not pleased with us. We can come home and kick the cat, put the dog out, and yell at our spouse. And we sit, pout, and feel terrible all evening and night, all because of some words. Your words are important as well; how do you come across once you open your mouth?

How do you characterize your own speech? Do you regularly choose positive, encouraging, comforting, kind, gentle, caring, and life-affirming words in your conversation with others? Or are you not aware of how you speak yourself? In most cases, we receive what we give out. If someone is having a bad day comes into the emergency room for treatment, and you are also in a bad mood, guess what is going to happen? I remember seeing a patient hit an RN one day, and I saw that same RN hit the patient. No one wins when you both are choosing to use harsh words. It often leads to violence and hitting; sometimes it can lead to a deadly outcome.

"Choices determine destiny" is my slogan that I coined several years ago and use on my business cards. It all comes down to your choice. You are the number-one "hearer" of what you say and the choices you make.

"Death and life are in the power of the tongue, and those who love it will eat its fruit" (Prov. 18:21, Holy Bible [NIV]).

It is my belief that nothing that we say goes unnoticed by the universal God or by our own subconscious minds. In fact, everything we do and say is noticed by the universal God; how you treat people in your care while they are in the hospital does not go unnoticed, and how they treat you as a nurse does not go unnoticed. Everything we say contributes either to the promotion of life of death. Cruel, hateful, and hurtful words can cause stress. Critical, faultfinding, and judgmental words can cause you stress. Rude, inconsiderate, whining, and complaining words can cause stress.

Millions of Americans find their harsh words amusing and entertaining (hateful and hurtful words); this is the kind of world we live and work in each day. Just take a look at our reality shows on TV, and you will see how we cut each other down with words and laugh about it. Is this really entertaining? And people may say, "Get a grip, it's just TV," but what we watch, we tend to become and mimic those values if we do it enough and we do not realize it. You come to work the next day after watching the TV show the previous night and try saying one of the lines you hear to get a laugh, but you hurt someone's feelings instead. Ridicule and mockery are made toward every profession and the people that work in them, even nursing. Some people have gone out and committed harm to others and themselves after finding out what someone said about them. Some of us work at high-profile companies, hospitals, and clinics where calling someone a stupid bitch, faggot, douche bag, or crazy asshole is an acceptable form of communicating in this society. Words can bring you down, and words can lift you up; words can cause you stress. For an example, receiving bad news from your doctor or attorney can cause increase stress in one's life. Words can also lift you up to places you've never been. Another example would be receiving word that you just won the lottery. Let your words be life encouraging, building up and not tearing down, positive and not negative.

> *Watch your thoughts, they become words,*
> *Watch your words, they become actions,*
> *Watch your actions, they become habits,*
> *Watch your habits; they become your character,*
> *Your character determines your destiny.*
>
> —Unknown

Choose carefully what you say, and I can faithfully say that stress will disappear in your life and in the lives of those around you.

CHAPTER FIVE

Stress versus Burnout

The worst days of those who enjoy what they do are better than the best days of those who don't.

—Jim Rohn

IN THIS CHAPTER, we will explore and distinguish the different between stress and burnout. These are some signs for RNs to look out for and to be aware if they appear present in your life. I will discuss what is considered burnout and what is considered to be stress.

DIFFERENCES BETWEEN STRESS AND BURNOUT

Stress can be characterized by overengagement, and burnout by disengagement.

Emotions are overreactive with stress, and they are blunted with burnout.

Stress produces an urgency and some hyperactivity, whereas burnout produces helplessness and hopeless. Stress produces loss of energy, and burnout produces loss of motivation, ideas, and hope. Stress can lead to anxiety disorder, whereas burnout leads to detachment and depression.

Stress's primary focus and damage is physical, whereas burnout's primary damage is emotional. Stress may kill you prematurely, as opposed to burnout, making one feel like life is not worth living. Stress can be characterized by the inability to find pleasure in activities, and burnout would be not being able to enjoy the activity. With stress, you usually find anger directed internally; with burnout, the anger is directed externally. Mr. Stress has unrealistic feelings of guilt, and with burnout, there is no guilt. With stress, one is more dependent; and with burnout, the person is more independent. Lastly, sleep deprivation is experienced by stressed-out, burned-out, and addicted people.

Stress can cause many of the same physical, psychological, and interpersonal/social symptoms as burnout. However, stress is different from burnout in that it is usually precipitated or brought on by quick situational instances, whereas burnout is the result of prolonged stress— when stressors constantly build up and pile up until the person is burned out. It is believed that job stress has a significant effect on ambulatory blood pressure, which leads to high blood pressure, which provides a partial explanation for the link between stress and heart disease. Stress and burnout are also associated with a range of psychological symptoms. Anger, violent, and depression are the most common psychological manifestations among stressed and burned-out workers; anger, which produces arguments, which produces violence, is probably the highest-reported incident in the workplace.

Gossip and more gossip among nurses tend to build until there is an escape, and sometimes it happens in the most unlikely places. Health-care professionals and especially RNs are trained to put the needs of others before themselves and spend each working day exposed to the emotional strain of dealing with people who are sick or dying, and who have extreme physical and/or emotional needs. Sometimes they reach a breaking point; the pain and strain are too much handle. This emotional strain, coupled with other stress factors, inherent in the health-care work environment, renders health-care professionals especially vulnerable to stress and burnout, especially in cancer units, intensive care units, emergency departments, and general medical-surgical units, which may produce more stressors if exposed for long period of time.

The highest rates of job dissatisfaction have been reported among nurses in hospice, nursing homes, geriatrics, and med-surgical units in hospitals. It has been reported that the rate of job dissatisfaction among hospital nurses has been estimated to be seven times greater than the average for all workers in the United States. One reason is because the majority of nurses work in a hospital setting, and most on a medical-surgical unit. By far, the most common source of stress and burnout among nurses is work overload brought on by inadequate staffing.

Communication theorist Marshall McLean once posed the following question: "If the temperature of the bath rises one degree every ten minutes, how will the bather know when to scream?" If you consider the environment a nurse works, and the setting, this hits the nail on the head when it comes to health care. When one considers the unhealthy lifestyle of their staffs, the overtime and double shifts create the bath from hell for the nurse. But you say, "It's all good," right? A good nurse should care. This is the expectations of the good nurses, yet nurses, even good nurses, soon realize that it is impossible to care for all people equally, and it is also impossible today to care for people adequately, given today's workload and system constraints. It is almost impossible for a nurse to care all the time, yet the expectations are there, not only externally but also internally, and many nurses who do not or cannot care enough feel guilty, stressed, or burned out.

TABLE 3

Here is what nurses encounter most of the time:

1 **Peer conflict**—"I don't like her or him"; "I can't stand that doctor."
2 **Schedules and shifts**—"I want off Christmas"; "I cannot work six days."
3 **Nurse manager**—"I don't like talking to him, he's a dick."
4 **Workload**—"I cannot get any help from anyone."
5 **Laboratory**—"Do we ever get labs here?"
6 **Patient care and teaching**—"I know I should, but I don't have time."
7 **Low performers**—"Why did they hire her? She doesn't work— too damn slow."

Sounds familiar? None of these quotes, I suspect, would surprise those in health-care industry today. However, this list is only part of the story; the real story is that the danger of burnout still exists, and it is a serious threat to the psychological welfare of health-care professionals and, in turn, those they serve, which include you, you, and you. I want to increase greater awareness of the effect, causes, and description of stress, fatigue, and burnout. Too often we hear the following statements made by nurses, physicians, and nurse's aides, and take them as part of the territory of working in a medical setting and not as symptoms that require vigilance. Let's look at a few more comments:

1 **Cynicism:** "This is just a paycheck. Nursing is not what it used to be. Nothing is going to change."
2 **Workaholic:** "My children need clothes and shoes, so I need to earn money and work more shifts than I'd like. But I don't mind, and I need to constantly check my texts, e-mail, Facebook, and voice mail even on weekends."
3 **Isolation:** "I really don't care for anything on the unit. The other nurses are nice people, but I am not getting close to them. I never discuss my work or personal life with any of them."
4 **Boredom:** "I am so damn tired of doing the same thing every day. When I am not killing myself, I am bored out of my mind."
5 **Depletion:** "I feel like I am getting nowhere on this job. I no longer feel the passion about the job as I did in the past. I am tired before I begin."
6 **Conflict:** "Everything seems to get on my nerves now. I fight with the patients, I almost hit one the other day, and I am no fun to be with at home. I also hate having to deal with patients' families because they always are asking too much from me."
7 **Arrogance:** "I wish I didn't have to deal with such dumbass coworkers. Also I wish the patients would just do what I tell them to do."
8 **Helplessness:** "I believe it's too late to try and change my situation. This is the workload I have to deal with, plain and simple. Also I think I am suffering from sleep deprivation. I have no time for family and friends."

Chapter Six

Reducing Stress

*Learn how to be happy with what you have
while you pursue all that you want.*

—Jim Rohn

Suggestions to Ease Stress: A Few Tips

FIRST OF ALL, know that stress is coming one way or another way. Talk to others nurses in your profession, especially nurses in different stages of their careers. Nurses with more experience will be able to relate success stories and will be able to call upon good memories of their time in the profession. Younger nurses will lack the experience, but their attitude can be inspirational. Nurses enter the profession because they want to make a difference and help others; it is nice to be reminded of these qualities in others and yourself. Here are a few tips.

❖ Keep a journal of your own memories and experiences. Take photos of your good things that day; sometimes a "bad day" can stay with us more easily than a "good day." Recording thoughts from better days will help remind you of why you enjoy your profession and what an impact you are making on people's lives. Focus on positive memories.

❖ Enjoy your time away from the hospital or workplace. The act of being a nurse is emotionally and mentally consuming. A great deal of energy is channeled outward; find the time to generate and rejuvenate more energy inward. It is OK to find some time for yourself when so much time is spent on others. It is OK doing things that you enjoy; you could do this: reading, exercising, spending time with a loved one, etc.

❖ Having sex with your partner and listening to your favorite's music. Mental exhaustion can take its toll on the physical body, so tension needs to be released.

❖ Exercise and meditation are two ways to relieve stress and gain more energy. Some people find benefit in lifting weights, bicycling, jogging, yoga, etc. Personally, I can say this has worked for me.

❖ Confiding in a close friend or a professional counselor can be highly beneficial. Talking about feelings and concerns is helpful, especially when a part of your own job is listening to the concerns of others. It can be emotionally draining for someone to regularly listen to other's concerns without releasing their own stuff.

❖ Take a class that focuses on the stressful nature of nursing and working in a hospital setting. The class may be able to offer suggestions and tips into handling the pressures of everyday nursing.

❖ Enroll in one of my seminars that I give on stress, burnout, and addictions in the nursing profession. Look at my website or contact me on Facebook or e-mail me for a schedule of a seminar coming to your city or state. Come and relax for a day and know that you are not alone; you will be joined by other RNs and nursing staff from all over who can proudly say, "I feel you." Smell the flower on the conference table, smell the coffee and relax, and celebrate a day from the job.

SOME STATS TO CONSIDER:

1   Workplace stress costs more than \$300 billion each year in health care, missed work, and stress reduction.
2   About one-half of Americans say that stress has a negative impact on both their personal and professional lives.
3   About one-third (45 percent) of employed adults have difficulty managing work and family responsibilities.
2   Over one-third (60 percent) cite jobs interfering with their family or personal time as a significant source of stress.
3   Stress causes more than half of Americans (65 percent) to fight with people close to them.
4   One in four people report that they have been alienated from a friend or family member because of stress.
5   Forty percent connects stress to divorce or separation.

Source: APA study, 2007.

PART TWO

BURNOUT

Chapter One

Is Your Hut Burning?

My life has a superb cast, but I cannot figure out the plot.
—Ashleigh Brilliant

IF I COULD use the analogy of a burned-out house, one would imagine how black and charcoal the walls and woods are, and you see entire rooms missing from the house; so it is with people who are burned out—they are not whole. Their feelings and emotions are burned and charcoal; they cannot feel anymore nor have compassion. They have lost the ability to feel and to care for others. They are hollow inside, missing entire rooms within themselves. Burnout is a very big problem. It affects the retention rate of nearly every hospital in the country. It causes nurses to feel exhausted and unable to care for their patients. If institutions were to change the work environment through decreasing the nurse-patient ratio, increasing nurses' pay commensurate with assigned responsibility, and valuing and recognizing the nurses' skills and knowledge, we wouldn't have to talk about burnout. I don't like talking about burnout. The reason being is because it is negative and reactive. I would rather talk about knowledge, which is positive and proactive. If we give the nurse the knowledge and power with appropriate staffing, autonomy at the bedside, and recognition of their value, we wouldn't have to discuss burnout in the first place. But the truth is, there are some nurses who are just burned out and probably should talk with someone about it. There are many nurses who are on another planet and totally disengaged in their jobs. There is a difference in engaged and disengaged nurses; disengaged nurses are the ones who show no compassion, don't mind hurting you with a needle or ramming a catcher in you, and show no sympathy toward your illness. And you can easily recognize the nurses by their expressions—stern face, no smile, but give you this look: "Why are you here?" And you begin wondering yourself, did I come to the right place? These RNs are totally disengaged from their jobs, patients, and workplace.

Anxiety, depression, burnout, and addictions can be serious conditions that undermine daily functioning and health. According to the National Institute of Mental Health (NIMH), anxiety, typically a normal reaction to stress, becomes debilitating when it becomes "an excessive, irrational dread of everyday situations." In a given year, approximately forty million US adults (eighteen and older), about 18 percent of the US population, are affected by an anxiety disorder according to the NIMH. RNs are not excluded from this number; the ability to make decisions, remember details, and act fast is an important quality to an RN.

PUTTING OUT THE FIRE

In an ideal world, it would be great if nurses did not experience burnout because it destroys creativity, decreases productivity, lowers the quality of job performance, increases opportunities for mistakes, and puts the public at risk because of poor judgment. The feelings of having to do better adds further strain on the nurse because a shortage in a stressful workplace adds to the degree of burnout. Burnout is most likely to occur in people who feel overworked and unappreciated already. It often occurs in hospitals where nursing is the profession used the majority of the time. When a person is burned out, they lose their mental and physical abilities, and often have conflict from lack of information; they deal with excessive workloads, boredom, job dissatisfaction, and having no rewards, and all this plays a major role.

In the long run, nurses are considered to be particularly susceptible to burnout. They are most likely to burn out first compared to other comparable jobs, since their jobs are typically stressful and emotionally demanding, and since nurses are repeatedly confronted with people's needs, sometimes very needy and various problems of all sort and suffering.

Paul Pruyser, from the Menninger Foundation, quoted, "Sooner or later, health-care professionals who deal with conditions entailing much suffering or pain discover that they have to perform a task for themselves in addition to discharging their obligations toward their patients." Somehow, nurses do not look at themselves that way or think about themselves very much. Making provisions for oneself is not easy, for the very fact that they may not feel in dire need of such restorative and equilibrating act. Sometimes this means that one's psychological state has already moved in the other direction, where insomnia, tiredness, weariness, brooding, and a wistful or mournful mood are present.

Nurses' attitudes can protect them from identification with the patients, at the same time allow for controlled and limited empathy for the patients. Nurses must learn to deal with separating their jobs and assignment and not take them home. Do not take them so personal; all of this and learning how to deal with the traps of patients' transference and our countertransference take an emotional toll on our lives. The person in jeopardy of burning out is not alone in suffering these types of ill effects. Others are singed by burnout and not affected as much. Those who receive care of services, coworkers, family members, and friends, all these people can testify to the costs that the person's burnout has had for them as well.

Stress generated in the workplace can permeate our private lives as well. It has wrecked a many of personal relationships. Many marriages have gone bad because one of the partners brought home workplace stress. It could start over something as simple as "you don't love our daughter or son," and then an argument starts that sometimes leads to talking about divorce. Then both of you don't talk, but pout and sleep in different beds, without talking to each other, or you don't answer your spouse's text; if someone tried to text, the other partner will not answer. It can affect all those relationships on which we depend for restoration and reconciliation. The costs of burnout are immeasurable, from the waste of a fruitful career that took a long time and much effort to establishing the effects on patients or clients who are the recipients of the caregiver's services. We see the results of ineffectual coping strategies or techniques. Burnout is a progressive and chronic state not visible or detected very early because it usually occurs in those strong, self-assured people who mask their weaknesses very well.

Let's talk a little bit about masking; do you remember all of your masked heroes in movies? They all wore a mask to hide their true identity. The same thing is true for health-care professionals, especially nurses; they pretend they are Superman or Wonder Woman, able to bend steel with their bare hands and all the time crying from inside. It could be the pain from a broken relationship, guilt from a past relationship, and the shame of hiding it each day from your coworkers. This has been the case in many professions; burnout among educators, teachers, counselors, and policeman is a growing problem. This phenomenon has been attributed to the inability of educators to meet the increasing demands placed upon them to educate the growing disparity between these high professional goals and actual accomplishments, which may fall short of these ideals. Nurses, who were once caring and dedicated, seem suddenly to be merely "going through the motions," devoid of any real emotional commitment to their patients. In essence, "burnout" reflects dissatisfaction with the workplace, domestic situation, living state, and/or political state. At one extreme, burnout forces us to change our jobs, city, or living circumstances; at another extreme, it triggers a death wish. In workplace terms, we have to be able to gain satisfaction from what we do. We have to be able to turn occupational effort into social or economic values that can provide us with the satisfaction that sustains our motivation. Upon reaching middle age, we awaken one day confronted by the possibility that we will share the fate of our patients or our parents. How frightening is that? And this leads to a need to reappraise our lives. It dawns on us that our omnipotence is illusory and that our nursing practice of medicine, which demands sympathy, concern, and technical judgment, is too much for us to bear as the major focus of our existence, especially when we are also distracted by small stuff on many levels. Richard Carlson quoted in his book, "Don't sweat the small stuff, because it's all just small stuff." In the grand finale, after we are done stressing out and burning out, it was all small stuff. We may still manage to empathize with our patients, but if a spouse, child, or parent complains about his or her own lot, we lose our ability to sympathize. Irritability, sleeplessness, and fatigue may indicate that depression has come to our door and "burnout" is knocking.

"High Expectation"

American nurses, whether they are from rural mountains of Tennessee or from high-tech New York State, all of them face expectations from their patients, from their own profession, and from the society at large that are utterly unrealistic on a day-to-day basis. They are demanded to be Renaissance men and women in an age when that is no longer possible; they are expected to be the ultimate healers, tech wizards, and total authorities on sickness and diseases. Such expectations add to a rising tide of murmuring of accusations directed at doctors and nurses, as well as a growing feeling of uncertainty among nurses themselves about the nature of nursing in our society. No wonder that—despite his or her prestige, salary, and power—the nurse physician today is a wounded healer. Who could live up to such a world of expectations without either crumpling or hiding behind the masks of Superman or Batman?

"Burnout" can lead to suicide or attempted suicides. When there is an absence of pleasure, as a psychological or physiologic event, it limits one's alternatives. One should anticipate pleasure in work, just as one has to experience or fantasize pleasure in lovemaking, or physical or other intellectual activities. One has to have a dream, a vision, in order to survive. We have to find that drug-free experience that will make the endorphins flow freely. Pleasurable events can come from more than just sex; we must expand our personal lifestyles or our patient experiences so we can allow ourselves to be involved with something larger than ourselves. We need religion or a renewed belief in our superpower as healers to provide a focus for our importance to our patients.

"Burnout" will come to all of us if we live long enough. It will have an effect on those around us who would be supportive, loving individuals. April, a nurse who recently quit her job, said, "Burnout is not the experience of having too much to do, but rather it is not having the energy to do things you know you can do and not enjoying the things you used to love to do." One must have some passion about what they do; passion is boundless enthusiasm. If passion is the experience of being alive in the moment, and that sense of life is characterized by commitment, happiness, and vitality, then burnout may be viewed as the absence of passion.

CHAPTER TWO

Signs of Burnout

Make rest a necessity, not an objective.
Only rest long enough to gather strength.
—Nadine Gordimer

#1 Your coworkers are tiptoeing around you.
If you find yourself becoming cranky and irritable with coworkers you used to get along with, it may be a sign of burnout.

#2 You come in late and want to leave earlier three out of five days.
You used to wake up in the morning excited for another day, but now every day you seem to dread heading into the office. Once lunch passes, you become a clock-watcher, counting the minutes to the end of the day.

#3 Your apathy has replaced enthusiasm.
You feel no motivation, feel no sense of accomplishment, and have no desire to be challenged. It's like "Whatever." Those who are burned out lose their motivation to perform, as well as their feelings of pride for a job well done.

#4 You've lost camaraderie with your coworkers.
You're no longer interested in the company parties, picnics, or event network. You used to go to lunch, go out for drinks, and participate in

other company functions, but now have no desire in socializing in or out of the office. "I just want to go home."

#5 You're feeling physically sick.
You always feel tired, feel exhausted, have headaches, feel tension in all your muscles, and are suffering from sleep deprivation. These physical signs are common indicators of job stress and demonstrate that this can turn into a real problem.

Those nurses who are experiencing high amounts of stress in their lifestyle need to always be aware of the idea of burnout potentially looming in the future. While the term "burnout" is often thrown around in discussion of stress, do you really know what it means and how it's caused? Let us look into the meaning and causes of burnout.

What is burnout? According to *Webster*, burnout is a state of emotional, mental, and physical exhaustion caused by excessive and prolonged stress. It occurs when you feel overwhelmed and unable to meet constant demands. Now, does that sound like a job description for a nurse? As the stress continues, you begin to lose the interest or motivation that led you to take on a certain role in the first place. Burnout has been known to reduce your productivity, zap your energy, and make you irritable, leaving you feeling increasingly helpless, hopeless, cynical, and resentful. Eventually, you may feel like you have nothing more to give. Most of us have days when we feel down, bored, overloaded, or unappreciated; when the dozen eggs we keep balanced in the air aren't noticed, let alone rewarded; when dragging ourselves out of bed requires the determination of Iron Man. If you feel like this most of the time, however, you may be flirting with burnout.

If constant stress has you feeling disillusioned, helpless, hopeless, and completely worn out, you may be suffering from burnout. When you're burned out, things seem dark, problems seem insurmountable, everything looks bleak, and it's difficult to muster up the energy to care—let alone do something about your situation. You might be suffering from burnout.

The unhappiness and detachment burnout causes can threaten your job, your relationships, your health, and your life. But burnout can be avoided. If you recognize the signs and symptoms of burnout in its early stages, simple stress management strategies may be enough to solve the problem. In the later stages of burnout, recovery may take more time and effort, but you can still regain your balance by reassessing your priorities, making time for yourself, and seeking support.

CAUSES OF BURNOUT

OK, so we have decided that being burned out means feeling empty, devoid of motivation, and beyond caring. People experiencing burnout often don't see any hope of positive change in their situation most of the time. One other difference between stress and burnout: while you're usually aware of being under a lot of stress, you don't always notice burnout when it happens. It kind of sneaks up on you like a vampire and sucks all your blood.

There are many causes of burnout. In many cases, burnout stems from the job or your home situation. But anyone who feels overworked and undervalued is at risk for burnout—from the hardworking office worker to the polished executive who hasn't had a vacation or a raise in two years, to the frazzled stay-at-home mom struggling with the heavy responsibility of taking care of three kids, the housework, and her aging mother. But burnout is not caused solely by stressful work or too many responsibilities. Other factors contribute to burnout, including your lifestyle, diet, and sleep deprivation, and certain personality traits. What you do in your downtime and how you look at your world can play just as big of a role in causing burnout as work or home demands. Do you view this world as a nice place or a horrible place to live and work? Do you view the government as cruel and evil, or do you view the government as help for the people? All of your answers can affect the way you feel and produce burnout and cause you not to perform well at work.

WORK-RELATED CAUSES OF BURNOUT

1   Feeling like you have little or no control over your job
2   Lack of recognition or rewards for excellent work
3   Unclear or overdemanding job requirements
4   Doing work that's repetitive or unchallenging

5   Working in a chaotic or high-pressure workplace

LIFESTYLE CAUSES OF BURNOUT:

1   Working too much, doing double shifts without taking lunch breaks
2   Being expected to be too many things to too many people
3   Being superman or superwoman, taking on too many responsibilities.
4   Not getting enough sleep, causing sleep deprivation.
5   Relationships issues, too many partners.

PERSONALITY TRAITS THAT CAN CONTRIBUTE TO BURNOUT:

1   Perfectionist tendencies; things must be a certain way—in a row.
2   Pessimistic view of yourself and the world
3   The need to be in control; my way or the highway
4   High-achieving, type A personality

CHAPTER THREE

Warning Signs and Symptoms

Work is either fun or drudgery. It depends on your attitude.
I like fun.

—Colleen C. Barrett

PHYSICAL SIGNS AND SYMPTOMS OF BURNOUT

1   Feeling tired, beat, and drained most of the time
2   Health problems, feeling sick a lot
3   Frequent headaches, back pain, muscle aches; take a lot of medications
4   Change in appetite or sleep habits, too much or too little.

EMOTIONAL SIGNS AND SYMPTOMS OF BURNOUT

1   Sense of failure and self-doubt; don't believe in yourself.
2   Feeling helpless, hopeless, trapped, and defeated
3   Detachment, numb feeling, lonely feeling in the world
4   Loss of motivation, not a self-starter

5 Increasingly cynical and negative view of everything
6 No satisfaction and no sense of accomplishment

Behavioral Signs and Symptoms of Burnout

1 Withdrawn
2 Isolation
3 Procrastinating, taking longer to get things done
4 Using food, drugs, or alcohol to cope
5 Taking out your frustration on others
6 Skipping work or coming in late and leaving early

Burnout Prevention Tips

1 Take a daily break from technology. Set a time each day when you completely disconnect. Put away your laptop or iPad, turn off your cell phone, turn off the TV, and stop checking e-mails.
2 Set boundaries. Don't overextend yourself. Do not commit quickly. Learn how to say no to requests next time. If you find this difficult, remind yourself that saying no allows you to say yes to the things that you truly want to do.
3 Adopt a healthy eating, exercising, and sleeping habits. When you eat right, engage in regular physical activity, and get plenty of rest to avoid sleep deprivation, you will have the energy and resilience to deal with life's hassles and demands.

Take Care of Yourself First

The concept of self-care is one that is emphasized in every book or article you read on preventing job stress and burnout. Self-care needs particular emphasis for health-care professionals, as they have been trained to put the care of others ahead of themselves. It is important for nurses to recognize that self-care is not equivalent to selfishness; rather, self-care is essential for energizing, restoring, reviving, and maintaining the physical and emotional stamina to manage stress.

Self-care involves several universal lifestyle habits, such as proper diet, exercise, rest, and regular health care. Maintaining a healthy lifestyle is vital to avoiding the physical effects of burnout. Individuals should also seek activities that will help them disengage from their professional routine and provide enjoyment; individuals should have effectively managed stress in a variety of ways, including mindful meditation, yoga, relaxation techniques, music, art appreciation, reading, writing, sports, hobbies, and volunteerism.

Self-reflection has been suggested as a way to remind oneself why he or she entered the health-care profession and what feels good about the job. Spirituality may help some individuals derive a sense of purpose or meaning in life and enhance coping skills, especially for health-care professionals who work in hospice.

SELF-REFLECTION AND LOOKING INWARD

A day with our feelings: Are your heart and mind on two different roads?

Have you ever taken a moment of your time to stop and think about yourself? Those of us in the human service or medical field always think about that special person and that special family we are serving, and this is the way it should be. Too few of us take enough time to pause to think about how we are living and whether our lives are really good. If we are to continue to commit our lives to serving other people, we have no choice but to pause, catch our breath, and think about our own personal lives. After all, each of us is a very important person.

How do you feel when your day is over and you come home? What are your feelings about the day? Do you feel a lot of stress? Do you feel good about your day? Or are you disturbed and completely burned out? Do you ever say, "What a hell of a day I have had!" How do I handle this when the day is over and I come home? How do I work off stress? Let me assure you that it isn't an easy thing to do. We must make a commitment to God, your higher power, or the universal God. "God, I have lived this day to the best of my ability, so let me rest in peace this night."

As we face painful situations, we should always work toward deepening the meaning of our lives. We should keep things in proper perspective and learn to let painful things go. Nothing is more meaningful to me than private time for meditation, to think about how I feel. Just letting go is so great, and it always encourages gentleness. Just don't try to be a perfect person, because no one can be. Yes, not even you!

Food for thought: to live a healthy lifestyle, just be yourself and take life as it is and your problems one at a time. As you think about your stress and problems, where do you go to release and dump the garbage?

So when I come to the end of a day, I can put my thoughts and my work away. I will have that feeling as I take my rest that throughout this day, I have done my best.

Yes, I promise myself to help any person that I find in need. And I have kept that promise, but I must agree that the one person I have not helped mostly has really been me. You can't take care of someone else unless you also take very good care of yourself.

Peace to you!

CHAPTER FOUR

World / Global Impact

*All that we are is the result of what we have thought. The mind is everything, what we think, we become.

—Buddha

THIS IS THE world of doctors and nurses, and the reality into which they are immersed from their nursing school to graduation. It is a world of disease-afflicted lives lined up person after person, room after room, in which the charge nurse and nurses seem to be the only ones spared. Hardly a minute's respite separates one heart-rending, gut-wrenching emergency from the next. And through this minefield of random misfortune walk the nurse as if guided by guardian angels, apparently unscathed. Who among us has not identified with the young cancer patient who is refractory to treatment and scared to death, or the midcareer professional deeply unresponsive and too young to have had this massive stroke, or the parents trying to absorb into their consciousness the sudden, accidental death of a child, or a young mother whose child just died from an asthma attack? Instead of the afflicter's "why me?" the caregiver frightened imponderable becomes "why not me?" What roll of the dice, what act of fate, what divine intervention preserves me from any one of these circumstances? What makes it possible for physicians, nurses, and techs to confront these patients and circumstances day after day with caring and therapeutic resolve and to walk the balance beam pole between the paralyzing fear of their own mortality and the numbness of emotional disengagement?

In each encounter, we see ourselves indifferent or separated from our patients' circumstances by the luck of the draw but believe at a subconscious level that we are somehow protected by some magical force. It's like wearing a medic arm badge in the battlefield.

The ability to do that depends on our ability to empathize with our patients, to see ourselves in our patients. And that, of course, demands that we confront our vulnerability and the statistical likelihood that we, too, will experience the misfortune of illness and its life-changing implications. Some say keeping it real, and others would say keeping it in perspective.

THE IMPACT OF BURNOUT ON NURSING

It has been said that one-third of nurses were dissatisfied with the interactions with their peers and their jobs; many reported interpersonal conflict with other nurses is a stress factor in and of itself, but the lack of a close working relationship deprives nurses of their colleagues as a source of support.

Relationship with patients can also be stressful for many nurses; if you lack certain people skills in dealing with the many personalities encountered on the job, you will have a difficult time, especially in settings that present unique challenges, such as oncology, critical care, emergency medicine, and mental health, which are also settings in which high levels of burnout have been found. Talking with patients and their families about limited treatment options and end-of-life decisions can be particularly challenging for nurses, especially given that many patients and families in this setting are frustrated, sad, fearful, and angry.

THE EMOTIONAL DEMANDS OF NURSING

The emotional demands of the nursing profession are well recognized. In 2002, the American Nurses Association surveyed nurses with the question, "How do you feel as you leave your job each day?" The most common responses were exhaustion, discouragement, exhaustion, and discouragement, and saddened by what they could not provide for their patients. Despite these prevailing emotions, little is known about how emotional demands relate to burnout. First, nurses represent the largest faction of health-care professionals, with more than 3.5 million nurses in the United States, and they are the frontline for direct patient care in hospitals. Second, job dissatisfaction and subsequent burnout have been strongly linked to nursing turnover, which has led to the nursing shortage that began in the late 1990s. This shortage remains ongoing, and estimates for the shortage by the year 2020 range from 340,000 to one million, according to a national survey. Some find that hard to believe; I find that hard to believe. Third and most important, the inadequate nursing staffing levels caused by excessive turnover have been significantly associated with nursing errors and poorer patient outcomes. Thus, enhancing job satisfactions and avoiding burnout is crucial to maintaining a high-quality patient care.

The term "burnout" originated in the 1940s as a word to describe the point at which a jet or rocket engine stops operating. The word was first applied to humans in the 1970s by the psychiatrist Dr. Herbert Freudenberger, who used the term to describe the status of overworked volunteers in free mental-health clinics. He compared the loss of idealism in these volunteers to a building—once a vital structure—that had burned out, and he defined burnout as the "progressive loss of idealism, energy, and purpose experienced by people in the helping professions as a result of the condition of their work."

Many use the term "burnout" today, and the definitions have varied since the time the word was first applied to humans. The term has been used to describe a mild degree of unhappiness caused by stress, as well as any degree of distress, from fatigue to major depression. The root of burnout is in the work environment, the grind, the constant toil, but because not all individuals working in a single environment will experience burnout, personal risk factors must have a role in making an individual vulnerable. These personal risk factors include certain demographic variables, personality traits, and opportunity. Let me explain further about opportunity, depending on your physical makeup and predisposition. Some people, whether male or female, are given certain privileges and promotions quickly, which produce another variable to whether they would be prone to stress out or experience burnout faster as opposed to someone not given the opportunity.

Stress can cause many of the same physical, psychological, and interpersonal/social symptoms as burnout. However, it depends if you are under one hundred degrees of pressure or four hundred degrees of stress. An example would be if you were always assigned to triage and the other nurse is assigned to a nonurgent minor care. Stress is distinct from burnout in that it is usually precipitated by isolated or situational instances, whereas burnout is the result of prolonged stress.

Work overload: By far the most common source of stress and burnout among nurses is work overload brought on by inadequate staffing. Lack of control or lost of control by staff. A sense of control, or autonomy, is important to nurses, and job satisfaction is greater when nurses, especially younger nurses, feel as if they have some control over how they perform their job in which most of them have no control at all; they just do whatever they are told to do.

Chapter Five

End Results of Burnout

Life is a great surprise. I do not see why death should not be an even greater one.

—Vladimir Nabokov

THE SPECIALTIES AREAS for the highest risk for burnout have been emergency department, critical care, and oncology. The rates of stress and burnout among nurses in these areas have been found to be higher than the rates among other health-care professionals, with approximately 60 percent of hospital nurses having burnout levels that are higher than the norm for health-care workers (according to American Medical Association). Other areas of concern are mental health, nursing homes, and AIDS units.

Those nurses who work in these areas experience high amounts of stress in their lifestyle and need to always be aware of the idea of burnout potentially looming in the future.

Nursing Shortage

The nursing shortage continues to be an issue that management and nursing schools has to deal with. It is directly related to the high turnover among nurses as a result of burnout. The shortage is expected to grow, and by 2020, there will be more than half million nursing jobs vacancies. Therefore, nurses need to be aware of the potential for burnout and how to avoid it.

What about Patient Outcomes

The shortage has left remaining nurses fearful of patient safety. I have spoken with several nurses nationwide who believe that staffing on their hospital unit is not sufficient to deliver high-quality care. Plus, most of them believe that the quality of care had declined over the past year and that they would not feel confident having someone close to them receive care in their facility. What do you think about that? If you are a student in nursing school these days, this is something to think about. Several studies have shown that decreased staffing as a result of burnout poses a serious threat to patient safety and outcomes. A survey of nurses found that errors in medication administration and treatment are in many cases perceived by nurses to be a result of the nursing shortage, but I believe it is burnout that stresses out nurses. When you are dog tired, exhausted, or high on some substance, it is easy to make a medication error. You can agree or disagree, but the facts remain. The primary goal in any setting is to stop the burnout cycle early by preventing the accumulation of stress. When implemented appropriately, preventing burnout is easier and more cost-effective than resolving it once it has occurred. Burnout that is addressed in later stages may take months or years to resolve fully. Thus, stress management techniques, seminars, and other interventions to ensure psychosocial well-being should be a priority for hospitals, health-care organizations, nursing institutions, and nursing schools, with a goal of preventing stress and managing it while in its early stages.

I believe there is one primary approach to preventing and/or coping with work-related stress and burnout. Given that the more than half of the factors in stress and burnout are related to the work environment, modifying the environment to eliminate the factors has the potential for the most success. However, it is often difficult to change organizational structure, which means individuals must make changes themselves. This is where time management comes into place; work on improving and creating a better work/life balance is to quantify the amount of time currently spent in each primary aspect of life—work, home, leisure, and vacation—and then determine priorities and assign preferred amounts of time for each aspect. I know it sounds like work, and it is, but overall, it will help alleviate stress and burnout in the long term.

PART THREE

ADDICTION SECTION

CHAPTER ONE

When You Want to Stop but Can't Stop

Choices determines destiny.
—Herbert R. Warner

IN A RECENT study, the Center for Disease Control and Prevention (CDC) reported more than thirteen million people used prescription painkillers nonmedically in 2010. I am quite sure that number has increased over the last four years.

Addiction, particularly prescription drug abuse, is a growing problem among adults and the nursing population. Supervisors and human resources representatives need to be objective and understand a person who may be struggling with addiction. These talks go best when you go in with a spirit of concern, care, and service. If there is anger or resentment about an employee's actions or failure, it's not the best time to confront the individual. You must consider this: most people who went to nursing school to become a nurse did it because they wanted to help others. Nurses are caring, compassionate, and loving, and they put the needs of others first. But what happens when the nurse is the one who needs to be cared for? What happens when a nurse falls victim to addiction? Just food for thought—and I will address these questions in the preceding chapter. But first, let's talk about what to look for when a nurse might be addicted.

WARNING SIGNS OF ADDICTION IN THE WORKPLACE

First and foremost, look for changes in performance, absenteeism, tardiness, inconsistent performance, lying, irritable, changes in appearance (weight loss or gain, change in grooming), isolation, smelling of alcohol, withdrawal tremors, nodding off at the desk, being revved, bloodshot eyes, dilated pupils, or constricted pupils. These are only a few—I am sure there are more signs; however, employers have a duty of care under health and safety legislation to protect the health of their employee. Employers should have an EAP (Employee Assistance Program) established in the workplace. Can anyone truly say that is happening in today's world? Is management taking an active role in helping these addicted nurses? Does your hospital staff take seriously the reports of someone needing help, or do they just follow the protocol by writing them up, giving them a suspension, or firing them? We will look more into management's irresponsibility and what can be done later in this chapter. Now let's talk more about addiction.

ADDICTION IS TABOO AMONG NURSES

Unfortunately, a nurse with an addiction is considered a "bad nurse" among their colleagues. Most nurses do not know what to do or how to handle it when they suspect a colleague has an addiction. Many nurses choose to remain silent about a nurse they feel may have a substance abuse problem. There is a certain bond or oath nurses have that states, "You don't tell on another nurse." Why? Because you never know when you may need a favor or someone to cover for you. Therefore, some of the reasons nurses may fail to report a coworker may include the following: they don't want to lose a friendship, they fear jeopardizing their colleague's nursing license, they would feel guilty, and they want to remain loyal to nursing and to their fellow nurse.

Addiction has an incredible power to lead people to do things that are so out of line with their normal behavior. It just makes you do dumb things without thinking about it. One disease that has, and still does, carry a stigma is addiction. Society has placed this stigma on anyone with the word "addiction" attached to him or her. It is slowly becoming an accepted disease in society. Depression used to carry a stigma, but it really doesn't anymore. Depression has been "accepted" as a true disease, therefore it does not carry that stigma anymore, and everyone you see will gladly tell you they are depressed. Four reasons that there is often added stigma for nurse addicts include the following:

1. Nurses are looked at as the caregiver, and therefore you cannot get addicted; there is added shame and guilt around the use of narcotics. That feeling of shame and guilt is multiplied when the nurse takes medication from patients. Nurses feel they are the caregivers, not the ones that need to be taken care of.
2. Nurses are more reluctant to admit they have a problem and seek help; they will be in denial for months before they realize there is a problem. They always have that fear they may lose their license if found out. And the stigma associated with a nurse who lost their license is huge.
3. Most nurses feel incredible shame because they violated not only their personal code of ethics but also their professional code of ethics. And then there are some nurses who don't give a damn about what people think. The next one is more distressing. Nurses are very proud of their profession, and when they fall to addiction, they fear that stigma of being the "addicted nurse" and believe it will follow them for life—in most cases, it does!
4. What nurses fear most is what their peers think about them if they are labeled as the addicted nurse. If their peers accept them the way they are, then they have less feeling of guilt and shame.

Registered nurses constitute the largest health-care occupation, with 2.4 million jobs, and about three out of five RN jobs are in hospitals.

But there are other departments in the hospital where you will find nurses working—and, yes, some working addicted. Here are a few departments and types of nurses.

TABLE A

Different types of nurses and departments:
    Critical care nurse
    Emergency department nurse
    Flight nurse
    Holistic nurse
    Home health-care nurse
    Occupational health nurse
    Preoperative nurse
    Per anesthesia nurse
    Psychiatric nurse
    Radiology nurse
    Rehabilitation nurse
    Transplant nurse
    Addiction nurse
    Developmental disabilities nurse
    Diabetes management nurse
    Genetics nurse
    HIV/AIDS nurse
    Oncology nurse
    Wound and continence nurse
    Infection control nurse
    Legal nurse
    Nurse informatics
    Dietitian nurse

CHAPTER TWO

Cost of Nurse Turnover

Can it be that man is essentially a being who loves to conquer difficulties; a creature whose function is to solve problem.
—Gorham Munson

HOW MANY JOBS have you had in the last three years? How many assignments have you gone on and left before it was over? Nurse turnover is a serious problem for health-care organizations. Nurse retention focuses on preventing nurse turnover and keeping nurses in an organization's employment. However, decisions about nurse turnover and retention are often made without the knowledge associated with the costs and benefits. How much does it cost to retain a nurse? What does it take to keep a nurse happy and loyal to her organization? This has become the concern of board meeting topics for many health-care organizations.

Concerns about registered nurse (RN) turnover become heightened during times of nurse shortages. These concerns originate from both noneconomic and economic sources. On the downside, there are concerns about the practicalities: retaining adequate numbers of RNs to appropriately provide safe care to patients and overburdening existing staff with increased workloads and demands that may bring about more staff turnovers. Now, there is another task of recruiting and attracting quality RN to fill vacancies. On the upside, there are concerns about the costs of turnover, the loss of funding capital, and the potential effects on quality of care. These concerns currently are being talked about by a wide array of individuals, from staff nurses to nurse managers and executives, and from hospital executives to health-care economists. Although it is logical to expect that turnover would adversely affect patient care, in reality, we know very little about nurse turnover in terms of quality of care and patient safety. But it is safe to assume that without adequate staff, patience care will decrease. Should patient have to pay for management ineffectiveness? Certainly not, cost of nurse turnover (or retention) may be difficult, but it would be no surprise if the aggregate costs of nurse turnover and vacancies were substantial.

DISRUPTIVE BEHAVIORS

Who would imagine **that one would find disruptive behavior in a hospital? Well, it may surprise a few and maybe not. Because you have addictions, burnout, and stress among nurses, disruptive behavior has become a major issue. Disruptive behaviors among health-care workers have threatened the safety and well-being of both patients and staff. The joint commission now charges health-care organizations seeking accreditation to address these behaviors and have in place a way of handling these situations when they arise. All members of the health-care team need to be knowledgeable about disruptive behaviors, period.**

Although disruptive behaviors have long been a concern among health-care workers, they have often gone overlooked, unchecked, or even worse, accepted as part of the system. By not addressing these behaviors, organizations silently supported and reinforced them. The good news is that these disruptive behaviors among health-care workers have recently come under increased scrutiny. The American Medical Association (AMA) has stated, "Personal conduct, whether verbal or physical, that affects or that potentially may affect patient care negatively constitutes disruptive behaviors." Disruptive behaviors include overt and covert actions; for nurses, this verbal abuse is frequently reported as coming from other nurses: using threatening or abusive language, making demeaning or degrading comments, humiliating someone in front of others, rolling eyes in disgust, ignoring the person, sending nasty e-mails, refusing to mentor, refusing to train, refusing to help others, throwing things, and even physically assaulting. Some of these behaviors are a result of mind-altering drugs; whenever you take something in your body to get high, it alters the way you think. Have you ever done something while you were under the influence of a drug that you would not have done if you were sober? Why? Because you are not in your right mind when the drug you took altered your reasoning. Have you ever woken up in bed with someone that you never thought you would sleep with? Have you ever done something stupid that you wonder what in the hell was I thinking? (Remember the movie *Hangover?*) You don't remember what happened to you while you were under the influence of some type of mind-altering drug. Remember the slogan, "Say no to drugs"—well, you still should say *no!* Addiction is linked to disruptive behaviors, and the more management is aware of it, the sooner you can help nurses who are struggling with it.

Chapter Three

The Addicted Nurse

If you don't like where you are, change it! You are not a tree.
—Jim Rohn

ADDICTION IN NURSING did not just start with the TV series *Nurse Jackie*. Addiction among nurses has existed for at least one hundred years. Historical research has showed that intoxication on the job existed even during the mid-nineteenth century when Florence Nightingale began her work. Drug addiction is a problem that is still present today. The America Nursing Association (ANA) defined an impaired nurse as one who has impaired functioning, which results from alcohol or drug misuse and which interferes with professional judgment and the delivery of safe, high-quality care. The ability to identify nurses who display early manifestations of being impaired could lead to an increased understanding of when to intervene through counseling and education. Identification of those at risk for addiction will allow for earlier intervention and possible prevention of nurses becoming impaired. Nurse managers need to know risk factors that lead to substance-related disorders and to discriminate between impaired and nonimpaired registered nurses based on those risk factors. Many nurses who become impaired are not identified until symptoms are already apparent and patients are at risk. Although impaired nurses may share common characteristics, they differ in development, progression, signs, and severity. Risk factors include heredity, family history, gender, psychological deficits, high stress levels, antisocial personality, ego weakness, and social cultural factors. The number of impaired nurses is difficult to estimate. Reliability of surveys is limited because of denial, fear of logical and occupational reprisal, and lack of agreement about the operational definition of impairment. Children of alcoholic parents appear to influence both the predispositions to abuse substances.

Drug addiction is a treatable disease. Some state nursing boards establish peer assistance programs to serve as confidential support groups for impaired nurses. These rehabilitative groups are designed to first intervene and then provide treatment referral, peer support, and assistance with reentry into the workplace. There have been some state licensing boards endorsing them because the emphasis is on helping chemically dependent nurses to recover rather than on imposing sanctions. I support this method and would hope that others boards and management organizations who are not controlled or regulated by some government entity would support it.

METHODS NURSES USE TO DIVERT DRUGS

Nurses are very clever when it comes to drug diversion. A variety of methods are used to divert drugs. First one is failure to administer medication to the patients, which was probably the most repeated one I heard when interviewing nurses. Nurses' mode of operation is to substitute saline for the medication and then use the medication themselves, which was reported as wasted, sometimes giving a partial dose. Also, another method is signing out medication that was not given and even stealing an entire of box of medication and destroying the sign-out sheet. That is when it is becoming a serious problem. So how does a nurse get that chance to steal an entire box of medications? Diversion or consumption of medications cannot occur unless there are opportunities to do so. Of course, the opportunity comes while they are at work. It was reported that most of the impaired nurses consumed drugs while on duty, and most of them used drug at least four times daily. It was reported that diverted medications were concealed by nurses on the person and most of the time in the wallet or the purse. Lockers were used less of the time, and the person's vehicle was used a small percentage of the time to conceal diverted medications. The third shift (11:00 p.m.-7:00 a.m.) was reported as easier to divert, and the medical surgical unit was identified as easiest unit to divert. When the opportunity presents itself, the nurse takes advantage of it. A nurse at risk who is experiencing a personal crisis and stress may carry the emotional and physical pain of the crisis to the workplace. If the high level of work-related stress compounds the crisis, the person may use drugs to alleviate pain (self-medication) in much the same way those analgesics are prescribed to alleviate patients' pain. The nurses use the drugs privately rather than with friends to protect their professional identity.

It has been reported that some nurses in crisis situations develop an obsession to obtain drugs quickly and frequently to reduce their pain. They will use any means deemed necessary to secure the drugs. The American Nursing Association (ANA) has cited attitude as a key factor contributing to the development of chemical dependency. What kind of attitude do you have? Do you know all the answers? Nurses have been trained to know the effects of many drugs. With this knowledge, they develop a false sense of security; nurses may feel that because of their familiarity with drugs, they are immune to the deleterious effects of using drugs and to the dangers of self-medicating because "I know how much to use." The process might resemble the sequence outlined below.

TABLE 3

1 **Thought process:** From a back injury to a migraine headache. "The pain is more than I can stand." Nurses remember how the drug made them feel and the euphoria that was felt, or they may depend on their knowledge of the effects of mood-altering drugs.

2 **Rationalization:** "I know I should not, but I am because I need relief. I will do it just this one time."

3 **Preparation:** A nurse devises methods to obtain drugs, often beginning with a legitimate source; when legitimate sources are exhausted, drugs are obtained by diversion. When diverting

drugs is no longer an option, nurse resorts to buying them off the streets.

4   **Experiment:** Different drugs are tried until the drug of choice is found.

5   **Decision:** The decision was made and the drugs was obtained, so problem solved. Wrong! It is only beginning; now your physiological need cannot be denied.

6   **Rationalization:** Eventually, the rationalization becomes "I got this, and I will handle it, I can stop whenever I want." (A false sense of security is present.)

7   **Consequences:** "I never ever thought this would happen to me." You got caught using drugs on the job, evident by random drug screen. Now you are facing the nursing board, and possible consequences could be suspension, revoked, fine, or whatever they think is proper.

8   **Acceptance:** "I have got to get myself together." Admitted that you do have a problem and have started the process to get yourself some help. Enroll in the EAP or a private rehab for nurses.

CHAPTER FOUR

A Different Kind of Addiction: Electronic Age—When Is Enough, Enough?

Do not go where the path may lead, go instead where there is no path and leave a trail.
—Ralph Waldo Emerson

ALMOST EVERY NURSE wears her cell phone on her as part of her medical equipment, second to her stethoscope. Nurses often are checking their e-mail while caring for patients or texting their significant other or child. Some studies have shown that mostly all US citizens with e-mail accounts check their e-mail frequently; this new research shows that a significant percentage of the population is addicted to their e-mail, and in more egregious ways than ever before. People are checking their e-mails while in the bathroom, bedrooms, bars, bus stops, doctor's offices, hospitals, and churches. I have even seen a man checking his e-mail at a funeral. It is not unusual to see a doctors or RN checking their e-mails while at work.

The constant connectivity that e-mail and smartphones provides means that people are becoming less and less capable of setting technology aside to focus on other things in life. I was out eating at a restaurant one day and saw this family of five sitting at the table, and all of them had their phones out doing something other than talking with each other and enjoying the meal. Because technology is so pervasive, it becomes nearly impossible to avoid; and the more access we have, the more often we choose to use it. As with addiction, e-mails have taken over our lives, and we must take control back, the same way as with any addictions, through support and treatment. Learn to say no to your cell phone—"You don't have to answer the text." Enough is enough, put down the phone! Patient safety is more important than trying to see who texted you.

IMPLICATIONS AND APPLICATIONS

Some suggestions if you are addicted:

1   Talk in private about a possible drug problem to your close friend or counselor.
2   Contact your company's EAP for help.
3   Consult with your church pastor or spiritual advisor.
4   Report possible drug abuse to a supervisor or manager.

ADVICE FOR MANAGEMENT:

Treat addicts with common courtesy and medical help instead of punishment or threat of jail; if a person is charged with a violation that stems from substance abuse, they are tried and thrown into jail with no treatment. Addiction is a disease, and it needs treatment. If you put a person in jail and don't treat the problem, the problem is still there when they get out. We need a better plan for nurses to get treatment because the legal system is not the answer. When it comes to drug charge offenses, there is more red tape for a nurse than it is for the ordinary Joe on the street; you can walk down the streets in some states and smoke marijuana because it is legal. A nurse's license would be suspended and fines paid if they were caught or admitted to any drug misuse. Allow them to use their Employee Assistance Program (EAP) if your organization has one and provide the resources to them to get help.

Advice for the Nurse

Improve Personal Lifestyle

1. Obtain adequate sleep—don't fall victim to sleep deprivation.
2. Ensure proper nutrition—avoid fast foods and enjoy a home-cooked meal.
3. Participate in regular physical activity—join a softball team or take up golf.
4. Identify and maintain priorities—do not run your life like a disaster.
5. Schedule adequate vacation time—it is important to schedule time off.
6. Participate in outside interests—volunteer at a homeless shelter.
7. Meditate; have sex regularly/or practice yoga—I have tried it; it can help.
8. Maintain sense of humor—that's the reason I married my wife.
9. Recognize limitations—we all have limits; learn yours.
10. Engage in self-reflection—in everything, learn perspective by reflecting.
11. Seek emotional support and practical assistance from family and friends.
12. Engage in spirituality—always recognize and thank your higher power.
13. Enhance communication skills—learn how to talk to people; be nice.
14. Learn gratitude—learn to be thankful for the small things in life.
15. Create a healthy supportive culture by being a healthier supportive person.
16. Remember why you became a nurse—before you can help someone else, you must first help yourself. Be well.

ADVICE TO NURSING LEADERSHIP AND ADMINISTRATION

Support from nursing leaders and administration is essential for job satisfaction. However, in my interviews with nurses, they do not have or perceive supportive leadership. In fact, most of them are dissatisfied with nursing management and administration because they do not listen to or address nurses' concerns or deal with nurses truthfully about decisions affecting their jobs. It has been reported that the lack of administrator and supervisor support has been a factor in high rates of burnout, stress, and addictions. Here are some quotes from nurses:

"OMG! I wish they would just get rid of those useless care plans (we normally do them in our head anyway). I dread writing narratives on each item. It is just so maddening and futile, and it is only there to show to JCAHO."

"All this paperwork! I usually spend one or two hours each day after my shift ends to complete the darn 'charting.'"

"There is never enough staff. Sometimes we nurses work without a single break at all in our ten-hour day. We are expected to not only be nurses but also be waitresses, cleaning staff, counselor, referee, and general gopher."

"Often I have to chase down doctors for signatures, questions, to sign off things that I feel they should have noticed when they were with the patient. I am not sure I trust some of them, to be honest."

"I am sick of not having enough supplies or the proper supplies. How do they expect us to work—they want us to be Mr. Gadget."

"Although it is sad, I feel like I have to consider another career for my own sanity."

"When management of health-care systems ever gets its act together and puts patient care first, I might stay, but for now, it seems to me it is all about money and getting by with as few nurses as possible."

This is a response from only a small number of nurses as you can see; however, there were many, many more quotes from nurses.

What Can Management or Health-Care Organization Do?

Strategies for Institutions/Organizations

I don't intend to attempt to try and tell management of health-care systems their job or how they should treat their staff, but I would suggest a few ideas to consider.

1. Sustainable workload—design a system where the workload is achievable.
2. Give nurses a feeling of choice and control.
3. Design a program of recognition and reward on a frequent basis.
4. Develop a sense of community within the organization (company picnic, etc.).
5. Management should treat everyone with fairness, respect, and justice.
6. Develop a culture where nurses feel valued and their work meaningful.
7. Have a confidential and well-equipped EAP available to everyone.
8. Elect a nurse to participate on the management team so they will have a voice.

This is only a small piece of the puzzle of putting this health-care system back on track. Obamacare is not the answer. Is it possible the government is not trying as hard to fix the problem, but is becoming part of the problem? With regulation on top of more regulations until the health-care industry is drowning in paperwork and nothing gets done until twenty years later. I know that there are many more stories out there that need to be shared. You are invited to tell me your story. I am currently working on a collection of stories told by people just like yourself who have worked in hospitals and health organizations, and know how the system works. I will feature the stories in the next book I publish. You can play a part if you wish. Send me your stories to this e-mail address: *Drwarner2010@yahoo.com* or go to my Facebook. And of course, you can find my contact information on my website or in this book.

I am closing this chapter with a copy of the Optimist Creed Modified, the Florence Nightingale Pledge, and the Serenity Prayer all found taped to a nurse's locker.

THE OPTIMIST CREED MODIFIED

I promise myself . . .

I promise myself to help any person that I find in need.
To be so strong that the troubles I find will not disturb my peace of mind
I will always talk health, happiness and prosperity to every person that I meet.
To make all my friends feel that there is something in them
To always look at the sunny side of everything and make my optimism come true.
To think only of the best, to work only for the best and to expect only the best.
To be just as enthusiastic about the success of others as you are about your own.
To forget the mistakes of the past and press on to the greater achievements of future.
To wear a cheerful countenance at all times and give living creature you meet a smile.
To give so much time to the improvement of yourself that you have no time to criticize others.
To be too large for worry, too noble for anger and too happy to permit presence of trouble.
So when I come to the end of a day, I can put my thoughts and my work away, I will have that feeling as I take my rest that throughout this day, I have done my best.

The Florence Nightingale Pledge

I solemnly pledge myself before God and in the presence of this assembly, to pass my life in purity and to practice my profession faithfully. I will abstain from whatever is deleterious and mischievous, and will not take or knowingly administer any harmful drug. I will do all in my power to maintain and elevate the standard of my profession, and will hold in confidence all personal matters committed to my keeping and all family affairs coming to my knowledge in the practice of my calling. With loyalty will I endeavour to aid the physician in his work, and devote myself to the welfare of those committed to my care.

The Serenity Prayer

God, grant me the **Serenity**
To **Accept** the things I cannot **change,**
Courage to change the things I can,
And **Wisdom** to know the difference.

EPILOGUE

S TRESS, BURNOUT, AND addiction will continue to be part of the nursing world; I am not that naive to think that there will be an answer one day to make the nurse whole. However, I do believe if one person at a time would care enough to start to make small changes in the health-care industry, then one day, perhaps we would not have to worry about the care we might receive in these facilities. It is my hope that health-care systems, managed-care agencies, nursing boards, and schools of nursing would look at this book and consider making a change in some way that would benefit nurses now and new ones to come later.

Nursing schools would be wise to teach new nurses or have them to read this book as part of their requirements. The more exposure, the better it is for the nurse to be aware of what lies ahead in the nursing profession. I know that there are more stories out there waiting to be told; let me be your conduit to telling your story. As I had mentioned earlier in this book, to consider sending your stories to me; everyone has a story, but everyone has not had the opportunity to tell their story. I already have a collection of stories from RNs who have shared their stories of adventure, trials, tribulations, troubles, heartaches, and the list goes on. Some have shared wonderful stories of recovery and victory from turning their lives around that was once headed in disaster. There are some wonderful nurses out there who have already helped and are helping their fellow nurses to change their lives and live a life free of addiction. Nurses helping nurses is a wonderful phrase to hear. Share your story; I am sure it will help someone else make it. E-mail your story to *Drwarner2010@ yahoo.com*. Names would be changed to protect your confidentially. It will help someone else realize that if you came through it, they will say, "I can do it too." And that is the whole purpose behind the second book—to reach out and be a resource for nurses to learn from and help each other. In conclusion, I hope this book will increase the awareness of the seriousness and detrimental effects of stress, burnout, and addiction among our nation's nurses. I pray that each person that reads this book will have a better understanding of what nurses go through each day on their jobs. I admire the work nurses do and desire that they would continue to do their best work, while in the best of health, while in the best working conditions and working for the best employers.

THOUGHT-PROVOKING QUOTES TO RELIEVE STRESS

"He who smiles rather than rages is always stronger."
—Japanese wisdom

"Yesterday is gone. Tomorrow has not yet come. We only have today. Let us begin."
—Mother Teresa

"A child's life is like a piece of paper on which every passer by leaves a mark."
—Unknown

"We all live with the objective of being happy; our lives are all different and yet the same."
—Anne Frank

"Never regret. If it's good, it's wonderful. If it's bad, it's experience."
—Victoria Holt

"There's never enough time to do all the nothing you want."
—Bill Watterson, *Calvin and Hobbes*

"There is more to life than increasing its speed."
—Mohandas K. Gandhi

"Life is not a matter of having good cards, but of playing a poor hand well."
—Robert Louis Stevenson

"Stress is when you wake up screaming and realize you haven't fallen asleep yet."
—Unknown

"Adopting the right attitude can convert a negative stress into a positive one."
—Hans Selye

"It is not how much we have, but how much we enjoy that makes happiness."
—Charles Sprugeon

"Being happy doesn't mean that everything is perfect. It means that you've decided to look beyond the imperfections."
—Unknown

"If you don't like something change it; if you can't change it, change the way you think about it."
—Mary Engelbreit

"Life moves pretty fast. If you don't stop and look once in a while, you could miss it."
—Ferris Bueller

"Don't cry because it's over, smile because it happened."
—Dr. Seuss

"Be yourself; everyone else is already taken."
—Oscar Wilder

"You only live once, but if you do it right, once is enough."
—Mae West

"Live as if you were to die tomorrow. Learn as if you were to live forever."
—Mahatma Gandhi

"I may not have gone where I intended to go, but I think I have ended up where I needed to be."
—Unknown

"I have not failed. I've just found 10,000 ways that won't work."
—Thomas A. Edison

"For every minute you are angry you lose sixty seconds of happiness."
—Ralph Waldo Emerson

"Choose a job you love, and you will never have to work a day in your life."
—Confucius

"A lie can travel half way around the world while the truth is putting on its shoes."
—Mark Twain

"Experience is not what happens to you; it's what you do with what happens to you."
—Aldous Huxley

"Do not go where the path may lead, go instead where there is no path and leave a trail."
—Ralph Waldo Emerson

"I'd rather regret the things I've done than regret the things I haven't done."
—Lucille Ball

"Nothing in the world is more dangerous than sincere ignorance and conscientious stupidity."
—Martin Luther King Jr.

"Old men are dangerous: it doesn't matter to them what is going to happen to the world."
—George Bernard Shaw

"Death may be the greatest of all human blessings."
—Socrates

"Man's rise or fall, success or failure, happiness or unhappiness depends on his attitude. A man's attitude will create the situation he imagines."
—James Lane Allen

"Work is either fun or drudgery. It depends on your attitude. I like fun."
—Colleen C. Barrett

"All that we are is the result of what we have thought. The mind is everything. What we think, we become."
—Buddha

"Can it be that man is essentially a being who loves to conquer difficulties, a creature whose function is to solve problem."
—Gorham Munson

"Choices determine Destiny."
—Herbert R. Warner

"A great man stands on God. A small man stands on a great man."
—Ralph Waldo Emerson

"Life is a great surprise. I do not see why death should not be an even greater one."
—Vladimir Nabokov

"You always pass failure on the way to success."
—Mickey Rooney

"My imagination functions much better when I don't have to speak to people."
—Patricia Highsmith

"Family members are members by birth, if we had to vote for members, there would be no family."
—Herbert R. Warner

"Be steady and well-ordered in your life so that you can be fierce and original in your work."
—Gustave Flaubert

"Time is our most valuable asset, yet we tend to waste it, kill it, and spend it rather than invest it."
—Jim Rohn

"Happiness is like a butterfly which, when pursued, is always beyond our grasp, but if you sit down quietly may alight upon you."
—Nathaniel Hawthorne

"The only good is knowledge and the only evil is ignorance."
—Socrates

"The name we give to something shapes our attitude toward it."
—Katherine Paterson

"Friends are people that need help, not people who want to help you."
—Herbert R. Warner

Book Summary

T HIS BOOK IS about the most common issues that confront a nurse on a daily basis. It can cause him or her heartaches, heartbreaks, and heart troubles. Stress is, by far, in my opinion, a leading cause of heart problems, sickness, and depression in this country. In this book, I talk about awareness in our hospitals, clinics, and emergency departments. Everyone should feel comfortable and be confident of the nurse treating you or your loved ones; we must also remember that nurses are also human beings with issues and problems like everyone else in this world. This book is also a valuable asset to any nursing student considering going to nursing school or college to study medicine.

In this book, we look at stress, burnout, and addictions as they relate to the working RN each day. I have worked in the ER alongside nurses who share their frustrations at their jobs, management, relationships, and personal problems. Nothing is left out or kept private; nurses share their most kept secrets of the job. Everything is centered on addiction, burnout, and stress. I have talked with and interviewed several different nurses from all over the United States, from Seattle, Washington, to Memphis, Tennessee, from Arizona to St. Croix, Virgin Islands. All share the same stories, the same issues, the same stress, and the same struggle with addiction and burnout.

In this book, we want to make nursing organizations, health-care corporations, and hospitals aware of the need to have seminars and resources for nurses that are hurting, and show some sensitivity to the RNs' needs, and know that they have families, children, and loved ones too, and they sometimes are in crisis. I have had the pleasure of working alongside RNs in the nurses' station, patient rooms, and even stayed at nurses' homes; I have heard their stories and complaints, and there is always that similarity within the story of betrayal, burnout, stress, and addiction. And they feel as if no one is listening or trying to hear them or feel their pain.

The world needs to be aware of how awesome our nurses are in their current working environment. The world should be aware of how much they give in terms of commitment, service, and sacrifice, especially our travel nurses, who leave their homes and go on assignments for three to six months at a time, and of course, the nurses who work in hospice and the emergency departments throughout our country. Our nurses work hard and, unfortunately, sometimes play hard. That is when the addictions start, affairs on the job, depression, alcoholism, divorces, and sometimes suicides. Several years ago, I worked at a hospital with a nurse who I thought had it together, very smart, good with the patients, very friendly, and had an outgoing personality. A person whom you loved to be around and share moments with, but one day, she found out her husband did something unthinkable by cheating on her; she could not handle the pressure or the stress of it, so she committed suicide.

Sometimes the RN is hanging on by a thread, and we need to be aware of it and treat her or him with some respect and give them some help when they need it. We should not have to wait to hear the news that a coworker has committed suicide because of the stress, strain, pressures, and issues on the job or their personal lives. Let's be proactive to notice the signs and symptoms and intervene before a tragedy happens.

INDEX

A

addiction
  alcohol, 27
  drug, 27, 72-73
  warning signs of, 66
alcohol, 29, 53, 66, 72
American Medical Association (AMA),
    60, 70
American Nursing Association (ANA),
    58, 72, 74
anger, 29, 34, 65, 81
anxiety, 20, 24, 28-29, 44

B

burnout
  causes of, 50-51
  definition of, 49, 58
  preventing, 53, 61
  signs and symptoms of, 48-49, 52-
    53

D

depression, 23, 25-26, 28-29, 33-34,
    44, 46, 58, 67, 93-94
disruptive behaviors, 70-71
drug abuse, 65, 77
drugs, mind-altering, 71

E

Employee Assistance Program (EAP),
    26, 66, 75, 77

F

Florence Nightingale Pledge, 81-82

H

habits, 32, 53
helplessness, 30, 33, 36